D1622929

BRODART, CO.   Cat. No. 23-233   Printed in U.S.A.

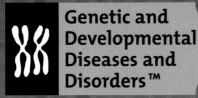

Genetic and Developmental Diseases and Disorders™

Muscular Dystrophy

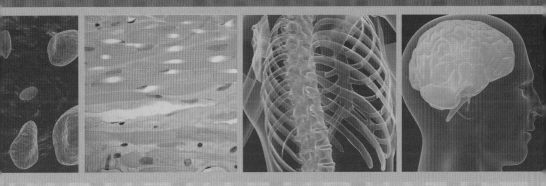

Paula Johanson

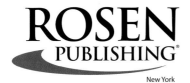

ROSEN PUBLISHING®

New York

For my children, with our own recessive and dominant traits

Published in 2009 by The Rosen Publishing Group, Inc.
29 East 21st Street, New York, NY 10010

First Edition

Library of Congress Cataloging-in-Publication Data

Johanson, Paula.
Muscular dystrophy / Paula Johanson.—1st ed.
    p.cm.— (Genetic and developmental diseases and disorders)
Includes bibliographical references and index.
ISBN-13: 978-1-4042-1850-5 (library binding)
1. Muscular dystrophy. I. Title.
RC935.M7J64 2008
616.7'48—dc22

                                                    2007040002

Manufactured in Malaysia

On the cover: Background: This micrograph image shows muscle tissue from a person who has Duchenne muscular dystrophy. Foreground: This photograph shows normal muscle tissue.

Contents

Introduction

There's a lot you can learn about muscular dystrophy (MD) that will be helpful. If knowledge is power, then knowing more about this disorder will help you have the power to improve your life or the life of someone you know who has been diagnosed with muscular dystrophy.

Muscular dystrophy is not a disease that someone can catch from another person, like the measles or a cold, so it's not infectious or contagious. It's a genetic disorder that gradually weakens a person's muscles. Muscular dystrophy is caused by missing or incorrect genetic information in the body's cells. The person's body is unable to make the proteins needed to build and maintain healthy muscles.

There are several types of MD. In the most severe forms, muscle problems begin when people are babies. The most common types begin to show in childhood and adolescence, though. Some forms of muscular dystrophy cause no symptoms until adulthood or middle age. A child who is diagnosed with MD will

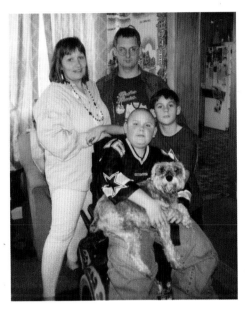

When the Norton family learned their oldest son, Michael, had MD, they joined the Muscular Dystrophy Association. Their whole family gets support because their lives are all affected by MD.

gradually have problems with walking, sitting up straight, moving his or her arms and hands, or even breathing easily. Other health problems can follow because of this increasing weakness. The heart can also be affected.

Although there is no cure for muscular dystrophy, researchers are learning about how to diagnose it early and treat the condition. Doctors have learned a great deal about how to improve muscle and joint function and how to slow the deterioration of muscles. Their goal is to help children, teenagers, and adults with MD live active and independent lives for as long as possible. Other research is looking at how to prevent muscular dystrophy from happening in the first place.

The History of Research into Muscular Dystrophy

1

Have you ever watched a crowd of people? Everyone moves differently. Some people walk quickly or run, while others walk slowly. A person who is older might use a cane for balance, and someone with a broken ankle might use crutches for a while. Some people move differently because of a disability.

Long ago, in many parts of the world, people who had physical disabilities were simply considered "crippled." But healers began to notice that some disabilities were different from others. Some physical disabilities can be treated or even cured. As modern medicine emerged, doctors began learning about one particular kind of disorder and how it was different from other health problems.

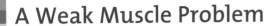

A Weak Muscle Problem

This disorder was usually noticed when a child who developed normally for the first few years began to stumble at around age five. The child may have begun having difficulty climbing stairs. Instead of walking naturally, the child might now waddle or walk on his or her toes instead of using the whole foot. The child might have difficulty getting up from a sitting or lying position or have a hard time pushing or carrying things.

There are lots of causes for any of these symptoms. Doctors became aware in the nineteenth century, though, that certain children had problems with their muscles becoming weak.

A Formal Medical Name

The name "muscular dystrophy" is used to describe this muscle weakness. The word "dystrophy" is based on two Greek words: *dys*, meaning abnormal or faulty, and *trophy*, meaning food or nourishment. Because people who do not eat nutritious food do not grow properly, doctors thought perhaps this weakness was due to faulty muscle nutrition. This was not the problem, though. These muscles were not being maintained, and they deteriorated because of the lack of a certain protein. Now the word "dystrophy" is used to describe this abnormal muscle weakness and wasting.

The first descriptions of muscular dystrophy (MD) were written and formally published in 1861 and 1868 by French neurologist Guillaume-Benjamin-Armand Duchenne (called Duchenne de Boulogne, 1806–1875). Some years earlier, Edward Meryon (1807–1880), an English physician, independently wrote a detailed description of the disorder. The name "Duchenne muscular dystrophy" has been assigned to the

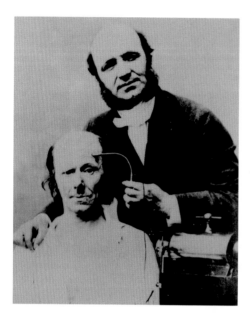

Guillaume-Benjamin-Armand Duchenne pioneered electric therapy and studied the physiology and diseases of muscles at Salpêtrière Hospital in Paris, France. This 1861 photograph shows him holding an electrode to a patient's head.

most common and severe form of this disorder. The other forms are called Becker, Emery-Dreifuss, limb-girdle, facioscapulohumeral, distal, oculopharyngeal, myotonic, and congenital muscular dystrophy.

The voluntary muscles are the muscles you control when you choose to move your body. They are also called skeletal muscles because they are connected to bones. MD affects the voluntary muscles. Over time, the weakness gets worse and different muscles are affected. In some forms, the heart and lungs can be affected.

There are many health problems besides MD that cause muscles to waste away and weaken. An infectious disease such as poliomyelitis, commonly called polio, may affect the nerve supply to the muscle. This disease is now rare in North America because of vaccination practices. Exposure to some chemicals or medicines can also cause nerve damage. Genetic problems can cause a variety of muscle conditions, too.

Myths and Facts

Myth: If someone in your house has muscular dystrophy, everyone nearby will get it, too.

Fact: MD is not contagious. It's caused by a mutated gene.

Myth: There's nothing that can be done to make muscular dystrophy any better.

Fact: Even simple acts such as eating sensibly, gentle exercise and stretching, and good posture can help keep someone with MD as active as possible for as long as possible. Medications can help, too. There is research being done to find gene therapy for a cure.

Myth: Only people who do bad things have children born with disabilities.

Fact: Doing bad things has nothing to do with it. Some genetic mutations happen randomly, whereas other mutations get inherited.

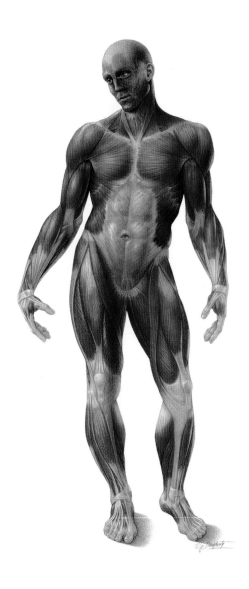

The skeletal muscles are under voluntary control. Shown in red in this illustration, skeletal muscles are attached to bone by tendons and other tissues, shown in white. Muscular dystrophy affects the voluntary muscles.

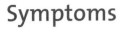

Symptoms

A child with MD may begin to waddle when he or she runs or walks. He or she may walk on his or her toes instead of using the whole foot; this swaybacked gait with the abdomen sticking out is called lordosis because it reminded watchers of a lord strolling in his robes. The calf muscles usually look enlarged, not because the muscles are growing but because the fibers are swollen, deteriorating, and being replaced with fatty tissue. This enlargement is called pseudohypertrophy.

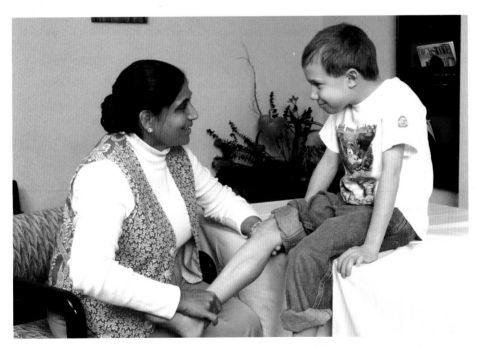

Daily exercise and gentle stretching are good for everyone's bodies. Physical therapy helps people with MD maintain the range of motion in their joints and delay the development of contractures.

GOWERS' SIGN

In 1869, Sir Richard William Gowers noticed that patients with weakness of the hip muscles had trouble getting up from the floor. He drew and described the way they moved: putting their hands on their knees or thighs and "climbing" up the body. Doctors often assess patients with suspected weakness of the hip muscles by having them perform this maneuver, now known as Gowers' sign. This is a classic finding in MD, but it can also be seen in patients with other muscle problems.

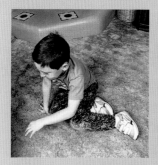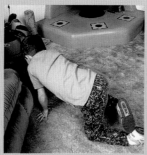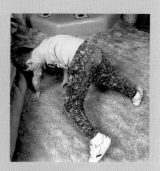

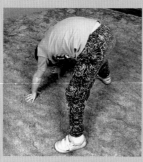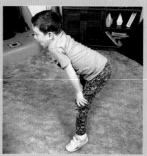

This boy cannot jump to his feet and stand up straight easily. He uses his hands on his knees to push his upper body upright. This is Gowers' sign of weak hip muscles.

Over time, the damaged muscles can tighten up into contractures and become unable to stretch. Then the limbs and joints can no longer move, making it hard or impossible for the person to walk, stand, or even use his or her arms and hands. Contractures can become disabling and painful and cause further weakness through immobility.

The muscle weakness from MD is usually symmetric, or the same on both sides of the body. The weakness is usually progressive, though this may vary among different forms of MD. Some types of MD begin at birth or early childhood and may progress rapidly to an earlier death. Other forms of MD begin later in life and are mild enough not to disable the person. In the most common form, Duchenne muscular dystrophy, the progress of the disease does not usually vary much and is relatively severe.

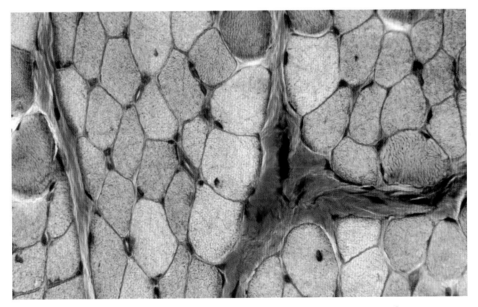

A slice of muscle tissue from a boy with Duchenne MD shows an increased amount of connective tissue *(pink)*. The muscle fibers vary in size from swollen to shrunken.

Understanding Neuromuscular Diseases

There are many diseases that affect the nerves and muscles, with a wide variety of causes and proper treatments. These are called neuromuscular diseases. Often what is learned about the causes or treatments for one disease can also be helpful for another condition.

The largest single effort to learn more about neuromuscular diseases is made by the Muscular Dystrophy Association (MDA), which was founded in 1950. The MDA works with more than two hundred hospital-affiliated clinics across America to provide comprehensive medical services to tens of thousands of people with neuromuscular diseases.

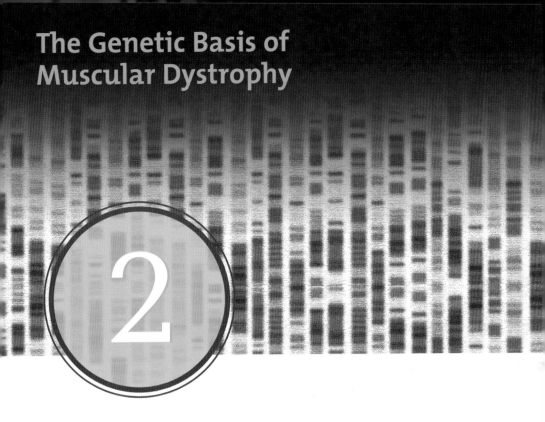

The Genetic Basis of Muscular Dystrophy

2

The cause of muscular dystrophy used to be a mystery. Doctors observed late in the 1800s that this disorder seemed to affect mostly boys and could run in families. It seemed to be inheritable, rather than caused by a virus or bacteria that anyone could catch, like chicken pox or strep throat. It didn't look like eating the wrong food or getting injured made it occur. More than a hundred years ago, doctors realized that MD is caused by a genetic problem.

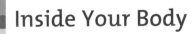 ## Inside Your Body

Your body is made up of parts that are too small to see. But if you put a sample of skin or blood on a slide under a microscope, you can

GATTCTGAACATGATACGTACTGGTGCCACTAGAACTGAACTCGAGAGGTACT

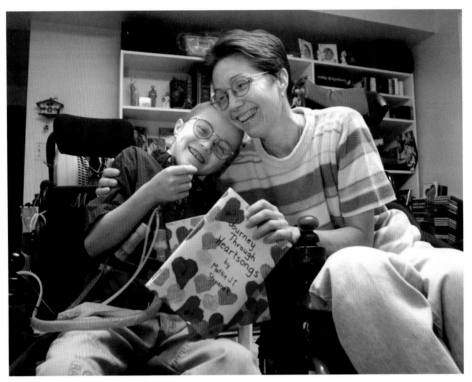

Mattie Stepanek, shown here with his mother, wrote best-selling and award-winning books of poetry. He had dysautonomic mitochondrial myopathy, a rare form of MD. Three of his siblings died from the disease, and his mother was diagnosed with the adult form only after she gave birth to her children. Mattie died a few weeks before his fourteenth birthday.

see these small parts like tiny bags or sections of an orange. Some fit close together like rooms in a building. The first people to see them were monks, who named them after a row of rooms where monks sleep, called cells.

Inside each cell are a nucleus and many proteins that the cell uses to do its work inside the body. Liver and spleen cells filter the blood, nerve cells carry messages, and white blood cells fight germs. Red blood cells carry oxygen. Muscle cells bunch up or straighten out so your body can move.

Cell Reproduction

After a few weeks or months or years, a cell will copy itself and split in two, a process called mitosis. During this copying, small pairs of rodlike shapes become visible. They're called chromosomes because they can be colored (*chroma* means "color" in Greek) by stains to be visible under a microscope. Inside these tiny rods are long, coiled molecules of deoxyribonucleic acid (DNA). DNA contains a series of four different smaller molecules over and over in various patterns. These

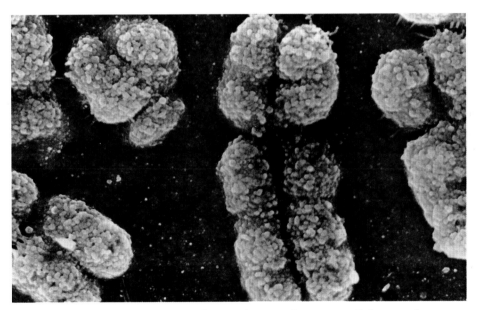

These chromosomes are making identical copies of themselves as a cell is making a replacement. The larger chromosome shown here is an X chromosome. The smallest is a Y chromosome.

chemicals make coded messages for how to make everything in your body.

Human body cells have twenty-three pairs of chromosomes. The twenty-third pair is the sex chromosomes that determine whether you are male or female: females have a pair of X chromosomes, males have one X and one Y. The other twenty-two pairs are sometimes called autosomes.

Cells inside your body's sex organs make eggs or sperm with twenty-three single chromosomes—a process called meiosis—so that an egg cell from a woman and a sperm cell from a man can combine to be the beginning of a new person. Everybody gets half their chromosomes from their mother, and half from their father. Everyone has a unique pattern of DNA, except for identical twins, who have identical DNA.

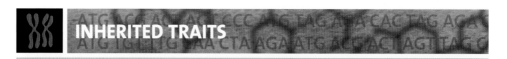

INHERITED TRAITS

The DNA molecules in your chromosomes carry genes, which tell your body's cells how to be certain types of cells and how these cells should work. You can inherit the gene for a trait that shows (a dominant trait), such as curly hair, from your mother or father. You can also inherit from one parent a recessive gene that doesn't have a visible effect because the other parent gave you a dominant gene on the matching chromosome of the pair. You may never know if you are carrying a recessive gene, such as the gene for blue eyes, unless you have a child with someone who also has that gene and the child exhibits that trait.

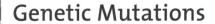

Genetic Mutations

Genes can also mutate, or change, so that the coded message in DNA might be missing one or more pieces, or part of the message might be repeated too many times. There could even be an entirely different part in the wrong spot.

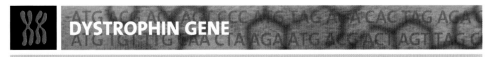

DYSTROPHIN GENE

A person's muscle cells are supposed to make a protein, dystrophin, that helps maintain the shape and structure of muscle fibers. If the gene carrying the coded message for making that protein is mutated, dystrophin may be absent or not work well. Mutations of the dystrophin gene on the X chromosome at position Xp21 cause most cases of muscular dystrophy. Researchers are still tracking down which mutations of some other genes on other chromosomes affect dystrophin and other muscle proteins.

Some genetic mutations are small and have mild effects that are not harmful. Some genetic mutations are severe. Many early pregnancies that end after a few weeks may be the result of a fatal genetic mutation.

Types of Muscular Dystrophy

There are nine main types of MD: Duchenne, Becker, Emery-Dreifuss, limb-girdle, facioscapulohumeral, distal, oculopharyngeal, myotonic, and congenital. Four of these kinds of MD, such as distal MD, are names describing a

CGATTCTGAACATGATACGTACTGGTCCACTAGAACTGAACTCGAGAGGTAC

group of related disorders caused by different genetic mutations with similar effects on the body's muscles.

Duchenne Muscular Dystrophy

Duchenne muscular dystrophy (DMD) is the most common kind of MD, caused by a mutation on the X chromosome. It is a recessive trait, which means females can be carriers of this gene but are usually not affected. Males have only one X chromosome and are therefore more severely affected if they inherit the mutated gene.

Duchenne MD is caused by a mutation of a gene that normally allows the production of the protein dystrophin. Without this protein, the muscles break down and a child becomes weaker. The level of a protein called creatine kinase released from muscle into the blood is elevated to dozens or hundreds of times the normal amount at first, then declines over the years.

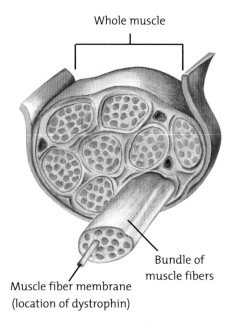

Whole muscle

Bundle of muscle fibers

Muscle fiber membrane (location of dystrophin)

Muscles are made up of bundles of fibers. Each fiber is surrounded with a membrane of proteins that help to keep muscle cells working properly. One of these proteins is dystrophin.

Symptoms usually begin to appear around age five as the pelvic muscles weaken and the calf muscles appear enlarged. Most children with DMD need to use a wheelchair by age twelve. Gradually the muscles weaken in their shoulders, back, arms, and legs. The muscles used for breathing get weaker as well. Eventually, a ventilator may be needed to assist breathing. The typical lifespan is about twenty years. Most children with DMD have average intelligence, but about one in three has some learning disabilities, and a small number have mental retardation. DMD occurs once in every 3,500 live male births.

Becker Muscular Dystrophy

Becker muscular dystrophy (BMD) is another distinct type of MD and is named after Peter Emil Becker, who first described

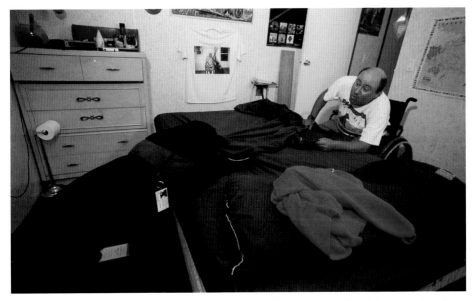

James Panuska uses a wheelchair. But he can make his own bed with a little help from his service dog, Hebert. Service dogs are beloved pets as well as trained helpers.

CGATTCTGAACATGATACGTACTGGTCCACTAGAACTGAACTCGAGAGGTAC

it in the 1950s. It is caused by mutations of the same gene that also causes DMD. These mutant genes do synthesize normal amounts of dystrophin, but the protein does not work properly. BMD causes similar symptoms to those of DMD but is overall less severe.

The onset of BMD is usually in the teens or early twenties, when the gait is affected by waddling, toe walking, and the development of lordosis. Weakness almost always begins in the legs and then affects the arms as well. Affected men may become confined to a wheelchair in their thirties. The heart may be the most affected muscle. Some intellectual impairment may occur, but it is less common than in the Duchenne form.

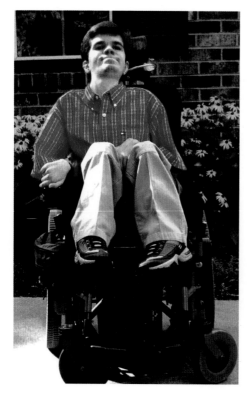

The Emery-Dreifuss form of MD can lead to difficulty bending the elbows, muscle weakness, and cardiac problems. A wheelchair is needed for some people with Emery-Dreifuss MD.

Death may occur in the twenties or thirties, but some men survive to middle age and beyond.

Emery-Dreifuss Muscular Dystrophy

Emery-Dreifuss MD is an uncommon type of muscular dystrophy. It was described in detail for the first time in the mid-1960s by Fritz Dreifuss and Alan Emery. Early recognition and proper treatment can be lifesaving. Inherited as an X-linked recessive trait, this is a relatively benign (mild) form of MD, but onset is in early childhood. The distribution of muscle weakness is different from DMD and BMD, affecting first the shoulder and upper arm muscles as well as the anterior tibial and peroneal muscles of the lower legs (which raise the foot). The main initial symptom is a tendency to trip over carpets and steps, rather than difficulty climbing stairs. Later on, the pelvic girdle muscles are also affected. Sometimes, a wheel-chair becomes necessary. Symptoms progress relatively slowly, and most affected boys live to middle age.

Muscle contractures develop early, before the muscle weakness is significant. The contractures usually affect the heel cords (Achilles tendons), causing affected boys to walk on their toes; the elbows, so that arms cannot be extended straight; and the back of the neck, making it difficult to bend the neck forward. There is no calf enlargement as in DMD.

Also, the heart is often affected, sometimes later in life, by an abnormal slowing referred to as heart block. Effective treatment may include inserting a pacemaker if the heart disease is severe. All individuals with this form of MD should be seen regularly by a cardiologist (a doctor who specializes in diagnosing and treating heart-related problems).

Limb-Girdle Muscular Dystrophy

Limb-girdle MD causes weakness to the limb girdle (major joints) of the shoulders and hips. There are nineteen or more

CGATTCTGAACATGATACGTACTGGTCCACTAGAACTGAACTCGAGAGGTAC

types of limb-girdle MD, inherited either as autosomal recessive or as autosomal dominant traits. All these types of limb-girdle MD affect both girls and boys, and are caused by mutations of any of several different genes. Each type of limb-girdle MD has some differences in progression of the disease. It's important to determine which kind of MD a person has, whether a type of limb-girdle MD or another MD affecting the muscles of the hips and shoulders, in order to treat it properly.

A female who has signs of limb-girdle weakness may be a DMD carrier who is symptomatic, that is, who shows some signs of muscle weakness. Usually a female who carries the gene for DMD on one X chromosome is not affected, but, rarely, she can manifest mild symptoms. As a carrier, she has a 50 percent risk each of having a son with the disorder and a daughter who is a carrier. A male who has limb-girdle weakness may have BMD, but a DNA test can tell for sure. A muscle biopsy will be done

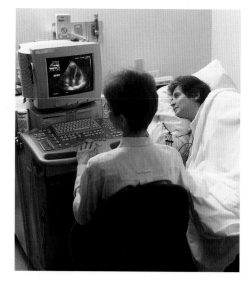

Heart function can be affected by limb-girdle MD. To monitor heart function, a technician is making an ultrasound image, called an echocardiogram, of this person's beating heart.

to allow studies of the cells and tissues. If both Duchenne and Becker types are ruled out, a diagnosis of one of the other muscular dystrophies may still be made.

The forms of limb-girdle MD differ in their age at onset, inheritance, and severity. Some forms are autosomal dominant, affect both sexes, and are inherited from an affected parent. Onset is generally after childhood, and these forms tend to be mild in overall severity, though the heart may be affected. Other forms of the disorder are autosomal recessive, so the parents are usually unaffected but some siblings of an affected child may also be affected. Onset is in childhood and tends to be severe. Many of the genes for these recessive forms have been identified through research studies. Most MD genes cause defects of certain proteins or deficiencies of muscle enzymes.

These are rare disorders in North America and western Europe, roughly twenty times less common than the superficially similar DMD. Limb-girdle MD is more common in Brazil and almost as common as DMD in northern Africa and certain Arabic communities.

Facioscapulohumeral Muscular Dystrophy

In facioscapulohumeral MD, there is facial weakness causing an inability to whistle or to close the eyes properly. The lips may appear to pout. Speech may become indistinct. The shoulder muscles around the shoulder blades (scapulae) may become weak or wasted. The shoulder blades become very prominent, like wings.

At the beginning, one side is often affected more than the other, unlike most forms of muscular dystrophy that cause symmetric weakness. The muscles that raise the foot are first affected. Tripping is frequent and running becomes impossible. As the disorder progresses, the pelvic muscles may become affected, causing a waddling gait and lordosis, and a wheelchair may become necessary. Hearing loss on one side is common.

CGATTCTGAACATGATACGTACTGGTCCACTAGAACTGAACTCGAGAGGTAC

This is the type of muscular dystrophy that varies the most from person to person, even among family members. Both males and females are affected, and this MD is inherited in an autosomal dominant trait fashion. The gene for this type of MD is located on the fourth chromosome. Onset varies from childhood up to age thirty. Some people may have only mild shoulder and facial weakness, or it may even go unrecognized. About half never have pelvic girdle weakness. Few become confined to a wheelchair, and many remain active their whole lives. In general, life expectancy is not reduced. Intellectual and heart function are not affected.

Distal Muscular Dystrophy

Distal MD affects mostly the muscles of the forearms and lower legs. There are several other disorders that can cause this pattern of muscle weakness, such as diseases of the spine and spinal cord or of the nerves serving these muscles.

From the beginning, there is weakness in the forearms and hands, noticeable as clumsy movements when using the

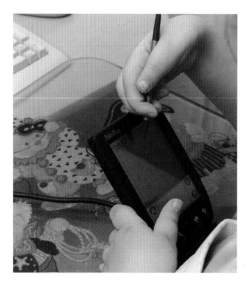

Contractures in the wrists, ankles, and other joints can impair a person's ability to do many simple, everyday activities. Contractures are more common with some forms of MD.

hands. When the lower leg muscles are affected, there may be tripping and difficulty in standing on the heels or toes. The muscles of the shoulders and hips only occasionally become affected. Lifespan is not affected, as the disorder progresses slowly. The onset begins after the age of twenty or thirty or even later. Both males and females are affected. This form is usually autosomal dominant, but some versions of distal MD are inherited in an autosomal recessive manner.

Oculopharyngeal Muscular Dystrophy

In oculopharyngeal muscular dystrophy, onset of the disorder occurs after the age of thirty. The eye muscles are affected and can sometimes cause uncoordinated movements and double vision. Later, the muscles of the upper face become weak, causing the eyelids to droop (called ptosis). It is common for the muscles of the neck and upper arms to be mildly affected. More seriously, it may become difficult to swallow, a symptom called dysphagia.

Most research of this autosomal dominant disorder comes from studies of French Canadian families with this form of MD. It can be traced back to French immigrants from 1634, and it also occurs throughout North America and Europe. A similar condition with earlier onset occurs in Ashkenazi Jews as an autosomal recessive gene. Recent research shows that many people with this form of MD have mutations of the genes in their mitochondria, the energy-producing "powerhouses" of the cells, rather than mutations in the nuclear chromosomes.

Congenital Muscular Dystrophy

When muscular dystrophy is present at birth, it is called congenital. These forms are usually inherited as autosomal recessive traits. At birth, some children seem to have no muscle strength, looking floppy or hypotonic. DNA study and a muscle biopsy help doctors be certain whether the

CGATTCTGAACATGATACGTACTGGTCCACTAGAACTGAACTCGAGAGGTAC

child has a form of congenital myopathy, or perhaps cerebral palsy, instead of a congenital MD.

Around half of all cases of congenital MD are due to a deficiency of merosin, a protein in the connective tissues around muscle fibers. Affected children are hypotonic and have joint contractures at birth, then later develop generalized muscle weakness and wasting. There is often difficulty in breathing. There may be some reduction in intelligence.

The other cases of "merosin positive" congenital MD are caused by a variety of rare autosomal recessive traits. In general, they tend to be less severe, and affected children usually learn to walk. One kind, Fukuyama congenital muscular dystrophy, is the second most common type of MD in Japan. It was described by Yukio Fukuyama in 1960. Affected children have generalized weakness and severe mental retardation, with few ever learning to walk. Calf enlargement is common. Many

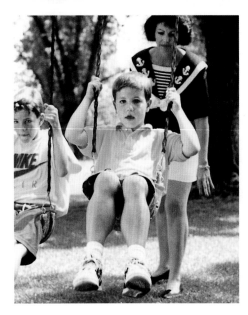

Some children with MD have enlarged calf muscles, a condition called pseudohypertrophy. This disorder is not from large, strong muscle fibers but instead is from swollen, damaged muscle fibers with extra fatty tissue.

also have epilepsy. As in DMD, the serum level of creatine kinase is grossly elevated at first and then declines over the years.

Myotonic Muscular Dystrophy

Also known as dystrophia myotonica and Steinert's disease, myotonic muscular dystrophy is the second most prominent form of MD and the type most commonly found in adults. Unlike any of the other types, the muscle weakness is accompanied by myotonia (delayed relaxation of muscles after contraction). It also causes a variety of problems in multiple systems of the body in addition to the muscle problems. When facial muscles are affected, eyelids may droop and speech may become unclear. As involuntary muscles become involved, there may be difficulty swallowing, bowel problems, heart problems, and uterine problems in females. Cataracts frequently develop, even in people as young as thirty.

While myotonic MD can affect males and females of any age, it is usually diagnosed by the mid-twenties. The severity of symptoms and disability vary widely from one person to another, even within a family. With each generation, the symptoms seem to get more severe and appear at a younger age, a tendency called "anticipation."

Myotonic muscular dystrophy is inherited as an autosomal dominant trait. It's caused by unstable mutations in either the myotonic dystrophy protein kinase gene on chromosome 19, or in the zinc finger protein 9 gene on chromosome 3. These mutations cause multiple copies of a short genetic message so that unaffected people might have between five and twenty-seven copies but a mildly affected person has at least fifty. Over time, a parent might have 150 repeats, a child 300 repeats, and a grandchild 800 repeats. It affects approximately one in eight thousand people worldwide. In parts of Quebec, Canada, the incidence is as high as one in five hundred.

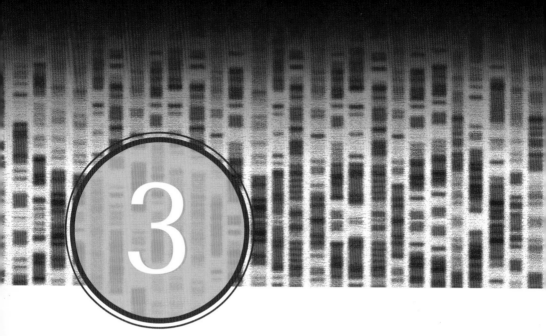

3

Being diagnosed with muscular dystrophy affects not only one person but also the people who care for him or her. When treating a patient with MD, health care workers are careful to consider the family as a whole. For them, the family is the patient.

Activity Helps

For children with MD, being physically active will keep the muscles functioning as long as possible. "Vigorous or violent exercise or strenuous calisthenics are certainly not recommended," says Dr. Alan Emery in his book *Muscular Dystrophy: The Facts.* "Moderate active forms of exercise do no harm and often have a beneficial psychological effect . . . The best advice is to encourage normal everyday activities wherever possible, supplemented with moderate exercise when this is appropriate and enjoyable." Adolescents and adults with MD should be physically active, too.

Swimming is an excellent exercise, promoting both strength and flexibility. It can also be a lot of fun. Children diagnosed with MD can learn to swim at a young age and can swim year-round when at all possible. Supervision by a responsible adult is needed.

Parents may worry that a child is being too active. If a child feels rested after a good night's sleep, he or she should

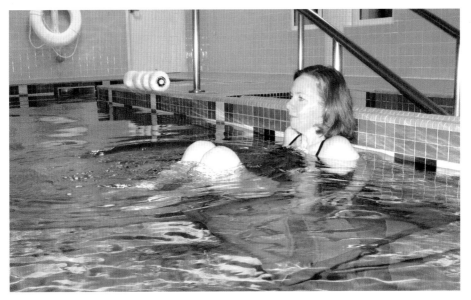

For many people with MD, swimming keeps the muscles flexible and toned. The buoyancy of the water helps in avoiding stress that can cause muscle injuries. Swimming is also relaxing and fun.

CGATTCTGAACATGATACGTACTGGTCCACTAGAACTGAACTCGAGAGGTAC

be able to participate in whatever activities that he or she enjoys and is able to do.

Physical Therapy

In addition to ordinary everyday activities, a person with MD should work with physical therapists to learn exercises that help the muscles and the spine. Many of these exercises will gently stretch various muscles. People with MD also participate in physical therapy sessions, where they practice walking normally with their feet flat on the ground and their bodies straight. Therapists can also help people learn to do everyday tasks, like brushing their teeth, dressing themselves, turning a doorknob, or operating a computer, when their muscles have become weak.

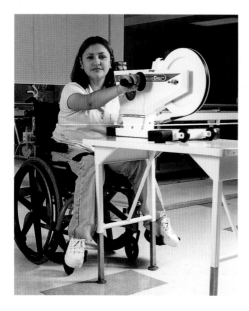

Physical therapy is practiced to maintain and improve movement of the joints. Special exercises improve a person's range of motion and delay development of contractures.

Passive Exercise

A professional physiotherapist should teach parents, partners, and friends how to do passive exercise of the affected person's arms and legs to keep the joints freely mobile. Gentle stretching exercises can be learned to delay (and sometimes prevent) the development and worsening of muscle contractures. These exercises should be a relaxing daily routine, and this gentle care will remain important even if the affected person can no longer walk.

Passive exercise is not a substitute for surgery if it becomes necessary. It is an effective way for a family to improve their lives, though. It costs nothing but time and attention, and it can be done while talking, singing, and listening to music or the radio together.

Speech Therapy

With some forms of MD, the muscles of the face and neck are affected and people have difficulty speaking clearly. Speech therapy can help people practice different sounds and improve their ability to speak clearly.

Some kinds of MD cause a person to begin having trouble swallowing, or dysphagia. Breathing can be affected, too. A speech therapist can help by teaching new breathing techniques or exercises that strengthen the tongue.

Physical Supports

People with the more serious types of MD eventually begin to have difficulty walking. Wearing leg braces can help to hold the weakened legs steady. These braces are made of hard

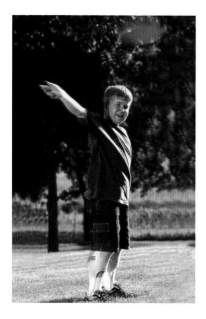

Lower leg braces offer support to help a person stand and walk on legs weakened by MD. Sometimes braces are worn while sleeping to keep a person's knees and ankles straight.

plastic that has bands strapped around the legs. In some cases, doctors believe that wearing braces every night during sleep will help delay contractures.

When people need more support, they can lean on a walker, a metal frame that may have wheels. If they become tired very easily, a motorized scooter cart or a wheelchair can be used part of the time. Eventually, it may become necessary to use a wheelchair most of the time.

Standing frames are sometimes used by people with MD so that they are not always sitting down in a wheelchair. The standing position can be good from an emotional point of view, and it can help so that one is not always in a seated position in a room of other people who are standing. A standing frame can also be good for promoting strength and blood circulation in someone who can no longer walk.

Surgery

Contractures that have become disabling and painful will not be helped by stretching and must not be forced. Some contractures can be partially corrected by surgery. Doctors will advise what to hope for when surgery is recommended. Sometimes the hope is to maintain or regain the ability to walk, to reduce pain, or to make it possible for an affected person to assist in being moved. Braces may be used after surgery.

Surgery may also be recommended if scoliosis (when the spine curves to the side) becomes severe. A rod may be inserted to straighten the spine, or pieces of bone may be put between vertebrae to grow in place and fuse the spine so it will not bend in that direction.

Drug Use

Many people with MD take pills daily for a variety of reasons. Cardiac drugs may reduce heart problems. Also, approximately 60 percent of Americans affected with Duchenne MD take steroid medications. On average, steroids can prolong the ability to walk for two or three years, delay the onset of cardiac and respiratory failure, and reduce the occurrence of skeletal defects. The side effects can be significant, though.

Obesity

When a person becomes confined to a wheelchair, the risk of obesity increases. This risk is particularly true for boys with DMD. Becoming obese makes it much more difficult to keep good posture in a wheelchair. Without strong muscles to maintain good posture, the spine may deform (scoliosis), and lung function may be restricted, which can affect breathing. Becoming obese makes it more difficult to maintain mobility, so contractures and other health problems become more severe. Also, it becomes much more challenging to help someone move, dress, or use the bathroom if the person is becoming obese.

Luckily, the increased risk of obesity seems mostly to be a matter of overeating and inactivity, just as it is for most people without MD. There doesn't seem to be any special added risk of obesity because the person has MD. Choosing a healthy diet will help a great deal to maintain a healthy body weight. If obesity does become a problem, dieting to lose weight or maintain it is well worth the effort. Maybe a family member or friend will become a "diet buddy" to improve his or her own personal health and for a sense of teamwork.

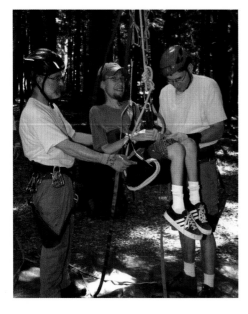

With assistance and teamwork, people with MD enjoy many physical activities, like technical tree climbing. Many groups sponsor exciting outdoor sports and indoor activities for people of all physical abilities.

Daily exercise to maintain strength and range of motion must be done and should be enjoyable to encourage a natural interest in ongoing, regular activities. Try a variety of activities and be willing to do new activities in new places with new people, as well as your favorites. Both choices—healthy diet and physical activities—are good for a family as a whole. A person with MD can take pride in helping family and friends maintain their own health as well.

Nobody's Fault

It's important for the parents and siblings of someone with MD not to blame themselves for carrying the gene or for not being affected. It is nobody's fault. Having one healthy child does not mean that the family's next child had to be disabled—the risk of passing on a genetic disorder is the same risk with each pregnancy. Also, at least 30 percent of cases of MD are new mutations that happen randomly. Someone with MD should not feel guilty if any siblings who are carriers plan not to conceive children—perhaps they will adopt, and adoptive children are real members of a family, too.

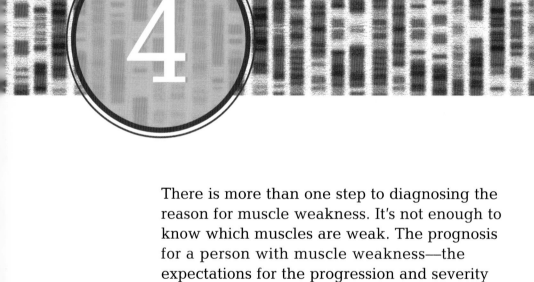

4

There is more than one step to diagnosing the reason for muscle weakness. It's not enough to know which muscles are weak. The prognosis for a person with muscle weakness—the expectations for the progression and severity of the condition—depends very much on the cause.

Muscular dystrophy is not the only cause for muscle weakness. Other causes include spinal problems, muscle inflammation, endocrine disturbances, infections, and certain drugs, particularly steroids. It may be a different inheritable condition. It is essential to get a precise diagnosis, not only to be able to help the affected person as much as possible but also to give the best advice possible for the health of other members of the family.

It's just as important to know which kind of MD a person has. Limb-girdle muscular dystrophy is not the only cause for limb-girdle weakness, for example. Limb-girdle weakness can be caused by other illnesses and also by other types of MD. These types must be ruled out, not only so the correct treatment will be known but so that family members can be given good advice.

Diagnostic Methods

The first thing a doctor will do is observe the person. How does this person walk or run? The person will be asked to sit and to get up again from the chair. Children with Duchenne MD often move in a certain way when getting up off the floor—Gowers' sign—which is easy to recognize. Climbing stairs is another activity to observe.

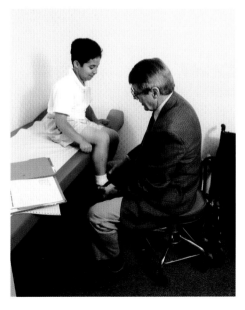

As well as doing many medical tests, doctors carefully observe a person with MD, noting his or her reflexes, breathing, movements, and balance, to see how the person is affected.

CGATTCTGAACATGATACGTACTGGTCCACTAGAACTGAACTCGAGAGGTACT

Sometimes the person will have small marks taped to the knees, elbows, and other major joints, and a video will be made of the person walking. Computer analysis can show small changes in the person's gait and compare them with videos taken on earlier visits.

The doctor will feel the person's muscles and test the reflexes. A test called an electromyogram, or EMG, will print a chart recording the electrical impulses in the person's muscles. Usually, this will show whether the person has a muscle disorder. Another test is a nerve conduction velocity test, which involves placement of electrodes on the skin to assess the speed at which electrical signals travel along the nerves. This assesses if the muscle weakness is actually due to a nerve disorder.

Muscle Fiber Damage

How can doctors know what's happening inside a person's muscles? They can't see under the skin to tell if enlarged calf muscles are healthy and strong, or swollen with fatty tissues replacing damaged muscle fibers. An X-ray doesn't tell much about muscles. Damaged muscle cells have leaky membranes that release an enzyme called creatine kinase into the bloodstream. When a person has less than the usual amount of a muscle protein called dystrophin, more muscle fibers are damaged and remain unrepaired. When a lot of the muscle cells are being damaged, there is too much creatine kinase in the blood, sometimes dozens or hundreds of times the normal amount if the person has Duchenne or Becker MD.

Doctors test affected persons and all family members for the amount of creatine kinase in the blood. It's easy to take a sample of blood, and it hurts no more than a needle prick.

Ten Great Questions to Ask A Doctor

1. Do you have any information that I can read about muscular dystrophy?

2. What do I need to know so that I can do the best I can to help?

3. How will having muscular dystrophy affect the rest of our family?

4. I'm really upset; is there someone who could talk with me, now or later?

5. What happens during the tests, and what are you hoping to learn?

6. What do I have to be careful about because of muscular dystrophy?

7. Is there any medication or other treatment that you recommend, and what is it intended to do?

8. Is there any exercise or physical activity that you recommend, and how will it help?

9. What should I expect for a year from now and five years from now?

10. Is there a self-help group for families with muscular dystrophy in this area?

This can help determine what form of MD a person has, and it can even alert doctors when someone is too young to have other recognizable symptoms yet.

Magnetic resonance imaging (MRI) is also used to characterize muscles. It doesn't hurt a bit. Any abnormality in size, atrophy, or fatty replacement can be monitored as the condition progresses. During an MRI scan, a strong magnetic field is created around the body, and radio waves are passed through the body to trigger a resonance signal that can be processed by a computer into either a three-dimensional picture or a two-dimensional picture like a slice through the body.

Biopsies are also done, which involves taking a small sample of muscle tissue. This can hurt more than an ordinary needle prick from a blood test, but a local anesthetic is used so that this test really doesn't hurt much. A biopsy is the best way to see exactly what is happening to the cells under the microscope. It's essential for diagnosing exactly what is causing the muscle weakness—which form of MD or other myopathy (muscle damage). Then the proper treatment can be done to help as much as possible.

 GROWING BIGGER

Some children are born with congenital MD and are affected from birth. But why would children with Duchenne MD, who show few effects when they are learning to move and walk, suddenly begin growing weak around age five? It's because most children are growing at that age. A small increase in the length of an arm or leg bone means a great increase in the volume of the arm or leg. The muscle is quickly growing bigger; without dystrophin, the muscle fibers simply can't maintain and improve themselves as they usually would.

X-LINKED RECESSIVE INHERITANCE

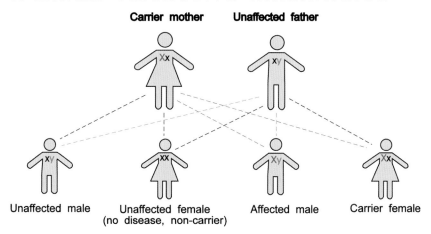

Carrier mother   Unaffected father

Unaffected male   Unaffected female (no disease, non-carrier)   Affected male   Carrier female

X = X chromosome with defective gene
x = x chromosome with normal gene
y = y chromosome

A child inherits an X chromosome from his or her mother and an X or a Y chromosome from his or her father. Inheriting a defective gene for MD makes a girl a carrier or a boy have MD.

DNA Testing

Samples of an affected person's DNA are tested for several of the known forms of MD. Family members will be tested to show who will also be affected or be a carrier of the gene. Family members will be advised of their risk of passing down the gene to future children.

About 30 percent of the time for cases of DMD or BMD, a normal gene mutated spontaneously in the egg or sperm cells of the parents. These mutations happen randomly, perhaps one in ten thousand egg and sperm cells.

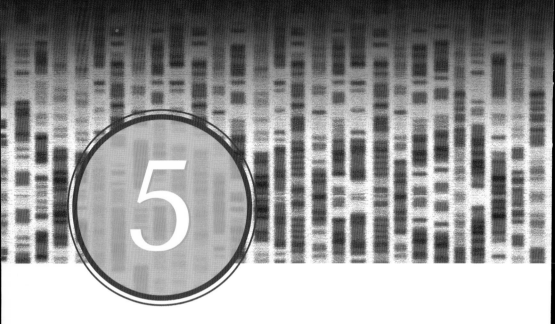

Different mutations of the Xp21 gene cause a variety of effects on the synthesis of the protein dystrophin. These mutations cause different forms of muscular dystrophy, ranging from the severe symptoms of early-onset DMD to the less severe Becker MD, which may allow affected men to survive into middle age, to forms that cause only relatively mild weakness in later life.

Mutations of other genes, such as the mutations on the fourth chromosome genes that cause facioscapulohumeral MD, are still being investigated for their effects upon dystrophin and the muscles.

It's very important to know which type of muscular dystrophy is affecting a person. Not

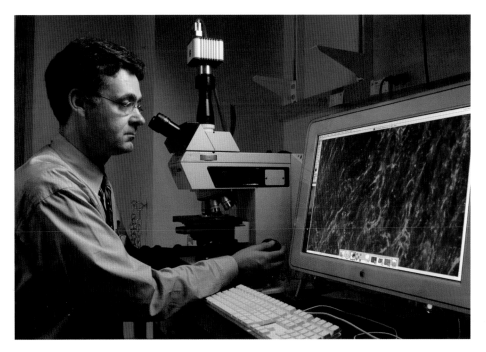

Researchers study the genetic causes of MD and other disorders of the nerves and muscles. They work to develop gene therapy, silencing the instructions of faulty genes, and cell transplants.

only will this make a difference for prognosis, treatment, and physiotherapy, but it will affect the family as well. For example, sometimes it's only after another family member has been diagnosed with facioscapulohumeral MD or oculopharyngeal MD that some adults learn what has been causing their own relatively mild symptoms. If a male has Duchenne MD, all of his daughters would be carriers of the gene. His sisters may be carriers of the gene and thus at high risk of having sons with DMD. Siblings of someone with an autosomal recessive type of muscular dystrophy may or may not be carriers of a mutated gene.

AFFORDABLE TEST

In 2003, Dr. Kevin Flanigan and other doctors with the National Institute of Neurological Disorders and Stroke announced a new DNA test for DMD that should make muscle biopsies less necessary. The new test, called Single Condition Amplification/Internal Primer sequencing (SCAIP), finds more than 95 percent of the mutations on the dystrophin gene that confirm DMD. Previously, multiple tests were required and were expensive and sometimes invasive, but they would still leave some 35 percent of affected children without confirmation of which mutations they had. The SCAIP test will also help researchers who hope to treat DMD successfully by identifying specific mutations and then tailor gene therapies to correct defects.

Mitochondrial Mutations

An increasing number of cases of oculopharyngeal muscular dystrophy are not due to mutations of the genes in the nucleus of the cells but to mutations of the genes in the mitochondria in the cells. That may seem like a tiny difference that doesn't matter, but it does. Mitochondria are important for producing energy inside your cells from the food you have digested, and you inherit mitochondria only from your mother. Men with this form of muscular dystrophy, which has its onset in middle age, can be confident that they have not passed on the mutated genes to any of their children. Women who have inherited the mutated mitochondrial genes would pass them on to all of their children. And all the siblings of someone who is affected with this form of MD should be tested as well.

Transplants

If surgeons can transplant a heart from a donor to someone who needs it, why can't they transplant muscles? It would actually be pretty difficult to move entire muscles into all the places where a person's muscles are weak. Everyone's muscle shapes are slightly different, for one, and the nerve attachments are too sensitive to cut and reattach properly.

In 1990, researchers began testing what happens if a few healthy muscle cells are injected into the muscles of a person with MD, hoping that the healthy cells would keep growing. Everyone's DNA is different, though. When cells or organs from a donor are put into someone else's body, they can be rejected by the body. The body's immune system can tell the difference. Drugs to reduce the chance of rejection are not always effective or good for general health.

Gene Therapy

What about transferring just the healthy gene for dystrophin into the nucleus of muscle cells in the body? This is difficult because the gene is too big to fit into the viruses used by scientists to bring genes into the nucleus of a living cell. It's the largest human gene we've studied. Cells are too small to be injected with hypodermic needles, but inactivated adenoviruses can enter living cells, just like the viruses that can give you a cold or the flu.

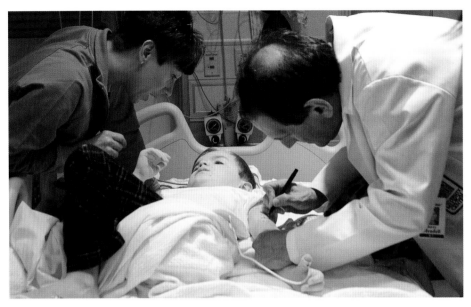

In this photograph, an eight-year-old boy is given an injection of genes for dystrophin into his bicep. If the procedure is safe and improves his DMD, the study will continue.

Instead of viruses, plasmids are used to bring genes into living cells. Plasmids are small DNA structures found inside bacteria. A French study was done in 2000 to see if injecting a tiny amount of plasmids with properly functioning dystrophin genes into a muscle would improve MD symptoms and muscle function. Researchers hope this may lead to a treatment that will preserve hand function and improve the quality of life.

For people with myotonic muscular dystrophy, their mutated genes are too large to function. Today, gene therapy is being researched that will use viruses to bring a small piece of DNA or RNA into muscle cells. The good genetic material will target mutated genes and mark them for removal by the cell's own machinery.

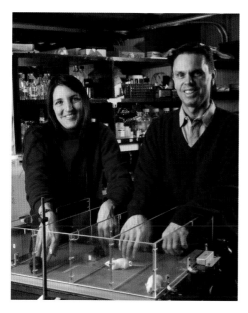

At the University of Pennsylvania, Elisabeth Barton and H. Lee Sweeney have given mice DMD and learned how to stabilize their condition. Sweeney hopes human trials will be even more successful.

Possible Hormone Treatments

Hormones are chemical messages that circulate throughout the body. A tiny amount of hormone will have profound effects, some of which are obvious, like growing taller or entering puberty, and other effects that are more subtle.

A hormone called insulin-like growth factor 1 (IGF-1) has been studied in mice that have been engineered to have MD. In these MD mice, gene therapy using IGF-1 improves muscle function, promotes regeneration, and prevents deterioration.

In addition, myostatin is a natural protein that restricts muscle growth. Drugs are being studied that inhibit myostatin's effectiveness and allow muscle regeneration in MD mice.

Utrophin is another muscle protein similar to dystrophin but is located on chromosome 6. There's more utrophin in muscles before birth than afterward. Even small amounts of utrophin make DMD symptoms less severe. Researchers are looking for drugs that could be circulated in the bloodstream to increase the action of utrophin without affecting other proteins or causing unwanted side effects.

For the Present

Existing treatments do prolong and improve the quality of life for people with many kinds of MD in many ways. Increased knowledge about MD and other neuromuscular disorders helps people understand both simple and scientific ways to promote health and wellness.

On a day-to-day basis, there are ways to improve the life of someone with MD that also improve the lives of other people. Activities, exercises, and good diet are important for people with MD and for their families and friends.

Making a building accessible to people using wheelchairs is not the only reason that schools and other public buildings install ramps alongside stairs and curbs, as well as powered doors that open at the press of a large switch. These doors and ramps make buildings convenient for people pushing baby strollers or delivering packages, as well as people who are older or have temporary injuries, such as broken ankles.

When public buildings and workplaces are accessible, being physically disabled becomes only a simple difference, not a limitation. After all, there are enough problems in the world that are hard to fix; making doorways wide enough for a wheelchair isn't really a problem. The Americans with Disabilities Act and similar legislation in Canada and Europe forbid employers from discriminating against someone who is qualified for a job and also is physically disabled.

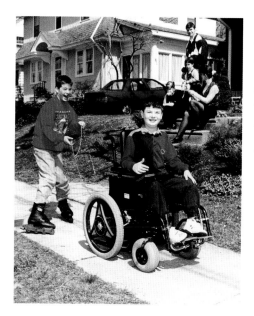

Improving life for people with physical disabilities improves life for everyone. Having MD or other conditions doesn't have to keep a person from being part of a family and a neighborhood.

Some people believe that this kind of progress—preventing discrimination and promoting accessibility—is as important to our culture as medical research is to find cures for MD and other conditions.

For the Future

There is no cure yet for MD. There is real hope, though, of effective gene therapy for the future, treatments that would reduce the effects of MD to prolong and improve the quality of life. This therapy will take years to develop and improve, but researchers are working carefully today. Even a fairly complete cure is not an unrealistic hope. Everything that scientists learn about gene therapy is another step toward that goal.

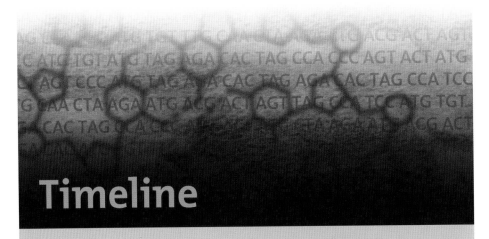

Timeline

1851

Description of muscular dystrophy by Edward Meryon.

1861

Muscular dystrophy is recognized as a specific disorder and described by Guillaume-Benjamin-Armand Duchenne.

1869

Sir Richard William Gowers draws and describes an identifiable maneuver for rising unaided from the floor when a patient has weakness of the hip muscles, now called Gowers' sign.

1950

Founding of the Muscular Dystrophy Association, a not-for-profit volunteer health agency.

1955

Peter Emil Becker describes a distinct type of muscular dystrophy.

1959

Serum creatine kinase (CK) first shown to be raised in patients and carriers.

1960

Yukio Fukuyama describes a form of congenital MD.

mid-1960s

Alan Emery and Fritz Dreifuss describe a distinct type of MD.

1983

DMD gene located on the X chromosome at position Xp21.

1984

BMD gene also located at Xp21.

1985

DNA markers available for carrier detection and prenatal diagnosis.

1987–1988

Gene cloned and protein product identified and named dystrophin.

1990

Injection of healthy growing muscle cells into a person with MD.

1990s

Gene therapy studies in animals. Protocols being considered for similar studies in humans.

1992

Robert Korneluk discovers gene for myotonic dystrophy type 1 located on chromosome 19.

1999

Gene therapy tested on a man with limb-girdle MD.

2000

Gene therapy using plasmids tested for safety on nine DMD patients over fifteen years old.

2001

Gene for myotonic dystrophy type 2 located on the third chromosome.

2003

Affordable, reliable blood test for DMD announced by Kevin Flanigan.

2005

Cardiac drugs (beta blockers and ACE inhibitors) recommended by American Academy of Pediatrics for children with DMD as soon as signs of cardiac dysfunction appear.

Glossary

autosomal dominant A trait that needs to be inherited on only one chromosome of a pair in order for a person to be affected.

autosomal recessive A trait that needs to be inherited on both chromosomes of a pair in order for a person to be affected.

autosomes All the chromosomes except for the pair that determine sex.

carrier A person who carries an inherited trait on one chromosome of a pair but is not affected.

chromosomes Small, rodlike packages of genes inside the nucleus of each cell that become visible when the cell copies itself and divides in two. Humans have twenty-three pairs of chromosomes.

congenital A condition present at birth.

contagious The ability for a disease to be passed on to someone else by close contact.

contractures Tightening and shortening of muscles, restricting movement.

DNA Deoxyribonucleic acid, a long molecule coiled up in chromosomes that carries the genetic code to create all our body cells and their functions.

dysphagia Difficulty in swallowing.

CGATTCTGAACATGATACGTACTGGTCCACTAGAACTGAACTCGAGAGGTACT

dystrophin A protein that maintains and repairs muscles.

epilepsy A brain disorder causing abnormal electrical discharges in the brain; may be mild, moderate, or severe; may occur in some forms of MD.

genes Small packets of DNA inside chromosomes carrying information on how to make our body cells function.

hypotonic Weak muscle tone in voluntary muscles, causing "floppiness."

infectious The ability for a disease to make someone else ill as well.

lordosis A distinctive way of walking on the toes without putting the heels down, swaybacked with protruding abdomen.

merosin A protein found in the connective tissue around muscle fibers. Deficiency in this protein causes around half of all cases of congenital MD.

mitochondria Small parts inside cells that contain their own genes and affect metabolism.

myopathy A disorder of muscle weakness.

pseudohypertrophy Enlargement of calf muscles because swollen, deteriorating muscle fibers are being replaced with fatty tissues.

sex chromosomes The pair of chromosomes that determine sex. A female has two X chromosomes, whereas a male has one X and one Y chromosome.

traits Inherited body conditions in genes, such as eye color.

X-linked recessive A trait inherited on the X chromosome that causes males to be affected with a disorder because the Y chromosome doesn't have matching genes.

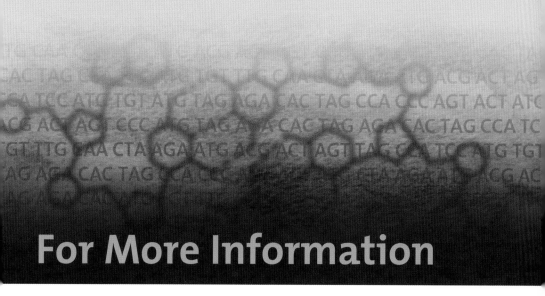

For More Information

Facioscapulohumeral Muscular Dystrophy (FSH) Society
3 Westwood Road
Lexington, MA 02420
(781) 275-7781 or (781) 860-0501
Web site: http://www.fshsociety.org
The FSH Society provides information, referrals, education, and advocacy programs about FSH MD and facilitates support groups.

International Myotonic Dystrophy Organization
P.O. Box 1121
Sunland, CA 91041-1121
(818) 951-2311 or (866) 679-7954
Web site: http://www.myotonicdystrophy.org
This international foundation is dedicated to improved management and treatment of myotonic dystrophy and supports patients with information and services worldwide.

Muscular Dystrophy Association—USA
3300 East Sunrise Drive
Tucson, AZ 85718
(800) FIGHT-MD (344-4863)
Web site: http://www.mda.org/main.html

CGATTCTGAACATGATACGTACTGGTCCACTAGAACTGAACTCGAGAGGTAC

This voluntary health agency fosters neuromuscular disease research and provides patient care at more than two hundred clinics funded almost entirely by individual private contributors.

Muscular Dystrophy Family Foundation
3951 North Meridian Street, Suite 100
Indianapolis, IN 46208-4062
(317) 923-6333 or (800) 544-1213
Web site: http://www.mdff.org
This organization provides services, resources, adaptive equipment, and home medical equipment to individuals with muscular dystrophy and their families to improve independence and quality of life.

National Institute of Neurological Disorders and Stroke
Brain Resources and Information Network (BRAIN)
P.O. Box 5801
Bethesda, MD 20824
(800) 352-9424 or (301) 496-5751
Web site: http://www.ninds.nih.gov/disorders/md/detail_md.htm
BRAIN makes contact information available for many associations interested in a variety of neurological and neuromuscular disorders.

OPMD in New Mexico
Health Sciences Center, MSC10 5620
1 University of New Mexico
Albuquerque, NM 87131-0001
(505) 272-6763
Web site: http://hsc.unm.edu/som/programs/opmd
The University of New Mexico hosts a research center and clinic for Oculopharyngeal MD, called OPMD, in New Mexico.

Parent Project Muscular Dystrophy
Executive Office
1012 North University Boulevard
Middletown, OH 45042

(800) 714-KIDS (5437)

Web site: http://www.parentprojectmd.org

This organization focuses on families with DMD and BMD and provides them with current news articles, research material, and information about medical treatment.

Web Sites

Due to the changing nature of Internet links, Rosen Publishing has developed an online list of Web sites related to the subject of this book. This site is updated regularly. Please use this link to access the list:

http://www.rosenlinks.com/gddd/mndy

For Further Reading

Burnett, Gail Lemley, Stephen D. Rioux, and Brenda Wong. *Muscular Dystrophy* (Health Watch). Berkeley Heights, NJ: Enslow Publishers, 2000.

Emery, Alan E. H. *Muscular Dystrophy: The Facts.* 2nd ed. Oxford, England: Oxford University Press, 2000.

Misheck, Barb. *A Wing and a Prayer: An Artist's Journey with Muscular Dystrophy.* Frederick, MD: PublishAmerica, 2007.

Muscular Dystrophy Campaign. *Thinking About You; DMD on the Ball; Same but Different; Everybody's Different, Nobody's Perfect; Hey, I'm Here Too!* Pdf pamphlet series for children. London, England: Muscular Dystrophy Campaign, 2007. Retrieved December 14, 2007 (http://www.muscular-dystrophy.org/care_support/daily_living_issues/education/materials_for_1.html).

Siegel, Irwin M. *Muscular Dystrophy in Children: A Guide for Families.* New York, NY: Demos Medical Publishing, 1999.

Stepanek, Mattie. *Reflections of a Peacemaker: A Portrait Through Heartsongs.* Kansas City, MO: Andrews McMeel Publishing, 2005.

Wynbrandt, James, and Mark D. Ludman. T*he Encyclopedia of Genetic Disorders and Birth Defects.* 3rd ed. New York, NY: Facts On File, 2008.

Bibliography

Curtis, Dan. *Bearing Witness: Luke Melchior.* Ottawa, ON, Canada: National Film Board of Canada, 2003.

Medline Plus. "Muscular Dystrophy." U.S. National Library of Medicine and the National Institutes of Health. June 27, 2007. Retrieved August 10, 2007 (http://www.nlm.nih.gov/medlineplus/musculardystrophy.html).

National Institute of Neurological Disorders and Stroke. "Muscular Dystrophy: Hope Through Research" July 19, 2007. Retrieved August 10, 2007 (http://www.ninds.nih.gov/disorders/md/detail_md.htm).

Stepanek, Mattie J. T. *Hope Through Heartsongs.* New York, NY: Hyperion Press, 2003.

Terpstra, John. *The Boys.* Kentville, NS, Canada: Gaspereau Press, 2005.

Ziegler, Tanya. "Accurate and Affordable Diagnosis of Duchenne Muscular Dystropy." National Institute of Neurological Disorders and Stroke. July 19, 2007. Retrieved August 22, 2007 (http://www.ninds.nih.gov/news_and_events/news_articles/news_article_dmd_test.htm).

Index

About the Author

For twenty years, Paula Johanson has worked as a writer and teacher. She writes and edits nonfiction books, including works on testicular cancer and HIV and AIDS. At two or more conferences each year, she leads panel discussions on practical science (usually biochemistry) and how it applies to home life and creative work. An accredited teacher, she has written and edited curriculum educational materials for the Alberta Distance Learning Centre in Canada.

Photo Credits

Cover (top) © Biophoto Associates/Photo Researchers; cover (inset) CDC; cover (background left to right) © www.istockphoto/Chronos Chamalidis, (two on right) © www.istockphoto.com/Sebastian Kaulitzki; p. 1 (left to right) © www.istockphoto.com/Chronis Chamalidis, CDC, © www.istockphoto.com/Sebastian Kaulitzki; pp. 5, 11, 12, 20, 22, 24, 26, 28, 31, 32, 34, 39, 43, 45, 48, 49, 51 © Muscular Dystrophy Association; p. 8 © National Library of Medicine/Photo Researchers; p. 10 © John M. Daugherty/ Photo Researchers; p. 13 © Custom Medical Stock Photo; p. 16 © AP Photos; p. 17 © Biophoto Associates/Photo Researchers; p. 21 © Time & Life Pictures/ Getty Images; p. 36 © Lon C. Diehl/Photo Edit.

Designer: Evelyn Horovicz; Editor: Kathy Kuhtz Campbell
Photo Researcher: Marty Levick